dedicated to the most
important element of
successful weight loss:

you

table of contents

Chances are, like most people, you've struggled with weight loss. You may have picked up this book because you're looking for answers. Or maybe you've heard about alli and want to learn more. Well, if you think this is about a miracle pill or that you won't be responsible for lifestyle changes, you should put this book back down.

The big question isn't whether a weight loss program will change your life, but will YOU? alli won't keep you from craving that extra

alli

slice of pizza or drive you to the gym when you need to work out. You'll be responsible for making healthy changes that are sustainable in the long run.

As you know, successful weight loss is difficult because it requires changing your attitude toward dieting, and changing your attitude about yourself. Changing the way you eat, the way you live, and only then, the way you look.

In this book, you'll learn from the experts about changing your behaviors, the biology of weight loss, the role of physical activity, nutrition, and more. You'll even hear from a famous chef who had to make a lot of changes of her own.

Remember, losing weight is a gradual process. And there may be times when you're not sure you can do it. But then you'll start to notice some changes. The energy to walk a little farther. A boost

alli

in confidence when your picture is taken. Even a tendency to eat healthier foods, simply because you enjoy them. And this is when you'll realize that losing weight is entirely possible.

It's up to you. If you're ready to lose weight without losing your mind, turn the page and begin.

[if you're ready, we're here to help you.]

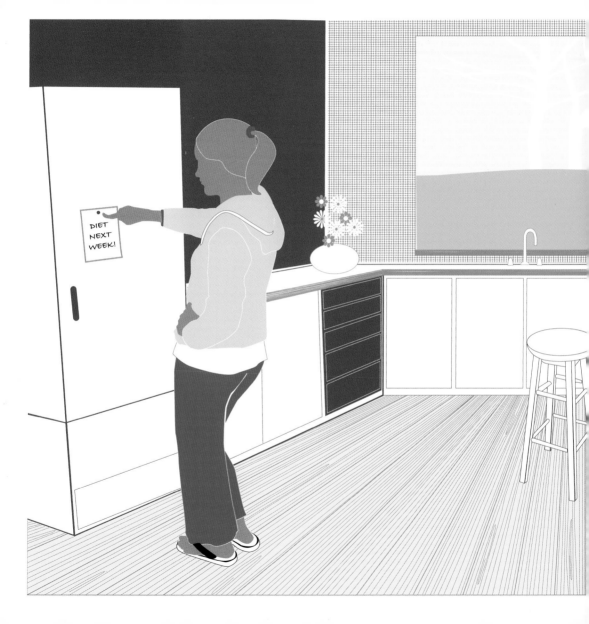

by **Gary Foster, Ph.D.**, the director for the Center for Obesity Research and Education and a professor at the Temple University School of Medicine

get out of your
own way

Solutions from an expert who has heard it all.

"People think losing weight is all about willpower. It's not," Dr. Gary Foster says. "It is also not about a moral issue. You have not been bad. You do not need to punish yourself with a life of white-knuckled deprivation."

[weight loss is about self care...

Foster has a doctorate in psychology from Temple University and is one of the nation's foremost researchers in the behavioral aspects of obesity. He has authored or co-authored more than 100 articles and two books on the treatment and causes of obesity. As a clinician, he has worked with thousands of people over 25 years, helping them to lead healthier lives.

"Weight loss is about self care," Foster stresses. "It is about taking time for self care. It's about changing your attitude, your behavior and your lifestyle."

alli

What prevents a person from doing this? All kinds of things. We don't have time. We're not supported. We can't stay motivated. We're tired; we're stressed. We've already tried every diet under the sun and nothing works.

In this section, Dr. Foster shares the six stories that he frequently hears. You may recognize yourself in them. If so, Dr. Foster's insights may be eye opening. It may not be easy, but you can have a stronger, healthier body and make it last.

Let's look at what's stopping you.

it's about **taking time** for self care.]

my life
is a game of
beat-the-clock

Every day is a race. It's not part of an exercise program. It's just the regular sprint to make sure everything gets done—family and work responsibilities under control, house relatively clean and organized.

Breakfast? That's a luxury I can't afford, not if I'm also going to get the kids fed and out the door on time. A drive-through mocha latte on the way to work gets me jump-started.

Lunchtime? Not about lunch. Not at my office. We're all too busy. I'd like to eat something healthy, but I gulp down a can of soda and polish off a bowl of instant noodles while firing off an e-mail or studying a spreadsheet.

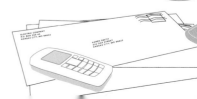

alli

I hit the wall around 3 every afternoon—time for a quick-charge sugar jolt to get me to the 5 p.m. finish line. An orange would be healthy. But oranges don't come in vending machines—candy bars do.

When it comes to making dinner, I've got a lot of things on my mind. Reviewing the reports in my briefcase. Helping the kids with homework. I don't have the energy or time to cook something. I end the day the same way I began—exhausted.

Being thin is easy if you have hours to spend at the gym or the money to hire a personal chef. But I'm not a movie star. I work hard. I take care of my family. I don't have time to eat healthy.

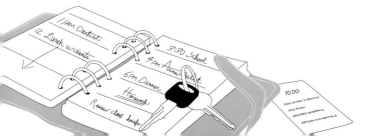

dr. foster weighs in:
don't make time for yourself—take it!

You have to accept that you are worth taking care of. You're taking on a new task here, and the bottom line is, it's going to take time every day. You have to dedicate time and make it non-negotiable. There are lots of ways to do this:

- Commit to leaving work on time at the end of the day.

- Go to bed earlier so you can wake up earlier and be physically active in the morning.

- Set aside 15 minutes for your own healthy breakfast.

- Delegate some of your responsibilities at home—so you can take the time to plan a week's worth of healthy meals, or take a relaxing walk.

alli

- **Stop spending money on vending machines and convenience store snacks.** Put it toward pre-packaged healthy meals from the grocery store.

- **Make meals on Sunday that you can freeze and reheat later in the week.**

- **Bring a bowl and some fruit to work with you.** Oranges and bananas in a bowl on your desk keep healthy options even closer than your vending machine.

The key thing is to make a plan and stick to it. If you plan and prepare, weight management becomes a lot easier. Of course, unexpected things always happen, and your routine will get thrown off. The important thing is to also plan ahead for the unexpected. Keep one or two healthy meals ready at home, and stock a drawer at work with healthy snack options. That way, no matter what curve balls come your way, you're ready.

i can't
stay motivated

I actually like starting new diets. It's a clean slate. A new beginning. All past failures erased. This time I'll do it. I'll be the new me in a month. Maybe sooner.

I cut out pictures from glossy magazines and plaster my fridge with images of thin, gorgeous women wearing the kind of cool clothes that I can never find in my size. I'll be able to get a whole new wardrobe in a month. Maybe even in two weeks.

I'm so psyched! I stock up on fresh fruit and vegetables. Skinless chicken breasts. Bottled water. I will no longer eat ice cream or cookies. No pre-packaged anything. Nothing salted or sugared or fried or buttered. I dig up my workout clothes. I will start actually using my gym membership three times a week. Maybe more.

alli

I sign up for spinning just to guarantee I'll go. I will be lean and toned. No more jelly belly! Good-bye arm jiggles! I will be bathing suit–worthy in a month. Maybe sooner.

I am unstoppable. I will not be deterred. I make it one day. Two days. Three days. One week. My arms are still jiggly. I ache. I'm sick of being hungry all the time. I'm cranky. I'm obsessed with pretzels. I'd kill for one. I want a life that includes cheeseburgers. A life where I'm not always frantic trying to fit in an hour at the gym. Where I don't have these stupid stick women mocking me from my refrigerator. I tear down the pictures and succumb to the bliss of salty, pre-packaged snacks.

I've failed again.

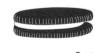
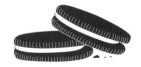

dr. foster weighs in:
small, cumulative changes last, sudden dramatic ones don't.

Lots of people say, "I go on a diet every Monday, and I get off track by lunch." They promise themselves they'll only eat 600 calories a day and spend an hour at the gym, five times a week. Nobody could maintain that kind of regimen. And who wants to live like that?

- **If you make a lot of drastic changes all at once, you'll set yourself up for failure.** With most people, if they start with the idea that they're going to the gym five times a week, and they only go four times, they see it as a failure. They won't see it as an 80 percent success. Developing healthy habits should be a positive process, and there's nothing positive about feeling like you've failed.

- **Don't look at it as a "diet"—a short-term means to a dramatic end.** Make changes you can live with, and think of them as part of a long-term, healthy lifestyle.

alli

- To effectively manage your weight, you need to make permanent lifestyle changes. That's a slow, gradual process. You can begin by setting specific and realistic goals. For example, in the first week, eat popcorn instead of chips; in the second week, be physically active 15 minutes more each day than you did in the past. Each week you can gradually build on your achievements. Focus on the process and not on a destination.

- If someone comes in and tells me they want to lose a lot of weight, I tell them to make goals in small, five percent increments. And, you don't have to cut your food intake by half to lose weight. You only have to cut it by a few hundred calories.

Find a balance. You can't obsess over every calorie, but you can't ignore your food choices, either.

get out of your own way

it doesn't matter
what i do,
the scale never **budges**

"

Rationally, I know the scale is just an inanimate object. A thing. But it has the power to make or break me some days. Depending on where that little red needle ends up, I can be either elated or full of despair. I know, I know—it's stupid, to put all that importance on a number. But I can't help it. When I'm on a diet, when I'm doing my part, I want proof that my hard work is worthwhile. That I'm worthwhile. So first thing every morning, I climb on. Well, almost first thing. I make sure I go to the bathroom right before, and I take off my rings. I hold my breath. I look down.

[i want proof that my **hard work**

alli

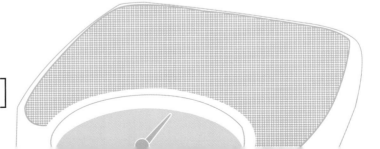

*I go from hopeful to angry and depressed in a microsecond.
How can I weigh half a pound more than yesterday?
Maybe the scale is broken. Maybe I stepped on it too
hard. I climb off and hop on again. Hold my breath.
Look down. The same. This is so unfair. I give up.
I've tried so hard. I feel like I could cry.*

is worthwhile.]

dr. foster weighs in:
learn to use your scale the right way.

Despite what you've probably been told, the scale is not the ultimate judge, especially if you weigh yourself more than once a day. You might gain a pound or two due to your menstrual cycle. Or because you ate Chinese food the day before and are holding on to a lot of sodium and water weight. The more often you weigh, the more fluctuations you'll see.

On the other hand, don't avoid the scale, even if you have not done as well as you would have liked. The scale provides a helpful reality check. Avoiding the scale means you are avoiding yourself and your commitment to good health.

alli

I advise weighing yourself at least once a week, preferably daily, but never more than once a day, and always under the same conditions—it's best to weigh yourself in the morning, after you've used the bathroom and before you get dressed. Remember, day-to-day fluctuations are normal. You need to track the scale through weeks and months to get an accurate assessment of your weight.

[day-to-day fluctuations are **normal.**]

quick **tip**

Developing routines makes it easier to stay on track.

my metabolism
is stuck **in reverse**

I used to be skinny. I have pictures to prove it. When I was younger, I could eat cake and french fries without instantly gaining five pounds. I didn't have to be constantly on guard, constantly denying myself. Now, my weight is a daily battle. Most days, I lose.

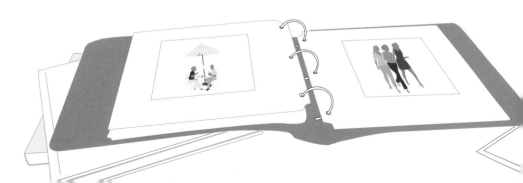

alli

I think my metabolism must have slowed down. Or stopped. Maybe it's gone into reverse. Is that possible? Anyway, my own body turned into a stranger. It went from gawky to doughy, even though what I ate didn't change that much. Maybe I used to work out more, but I'm still on the go, all day long.

[my **weight** is a daily battle.]

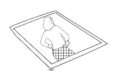

get out of your own way

quick **tip**

You are worth it. Believing that you are worth taking care of makes it easier to stay focused.

dr. foster weighs in:
keeping active helps keep your metabolism strong.

Yes, your metabolism, the rate you burn calories, does slow down a bit as you age. But that's related to losing muscle mass, not just a result of getting older. Building muscles by staying physically active can offset the small metabolic decline that comes with aging.

And it's important to know just how great physical activity is for your mind, as well as your body. Research shows that even moderate activity can help improve your mood and help prevent serious conditions like diabetes and heart disease. Additionally, all physical activity, from walking to watering flowers, burns calories.

alli

When I talk to people, I ask them what level of physical activity they feel comfortable doing. For a good 90 percent of the population, it's walking. Start small. Walk for 10 minutes. Even five. Your goal at first is to find a sustainable activity plan that works for you. Later, you can add muscle-building activities like Pilates, resistance bands or weightlifting.

Some people I've met think their metabolism is the only reason they are struggling with their weight. It's not. Weight loss involves a combination of factors. And my best advice is to focus on what you can control: sustaining healthy eating and activity habits.

[find an **activity** plan that works for you.]

i but hardly eat all day

I honestly don't understand why I am overweight. I shouldn't be. I never have three full meals a day. For breakfast I have black coffee and maybe a piece of toast, or half a muffin.

Lunch is normally some yogurt and a few crackers. I keep some candy on my desk, just in case my blood sugar drops, but I swear, I rarely touch it. If my colleagues and I go out after work, I never order appetizers. Or if I do, I'll share one.

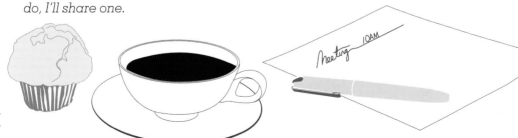

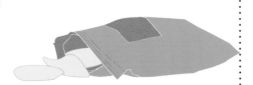

When I get home from work, I make sure my kids have a snack, usually chips or some cookies. As much as I would love to indulge with them, I do limit myself to only a few bites here and there. I make dinner, but I don't really sit down to eat it. I nibble while I'm cooking and clean up what gets left on the plates. It only adds up to a few bites.

So I barely eat all day. Yet I never lose a pound. It just doesn't add up.

get out of your own way

quick **tip**

Sometimes people think they can track their eating habits just as well in their heads. **Try writing everything down, and you will surprise yourself.**

dr. foster weighs in:

write on.

Most of us, whether we're overweight or not, vastly underestimate how much we eat. I ask my patients to keep a food journal. To write down every single thing they eat, and how many calories it has.

That can be hard at first, because you're constantly looking up calorie counts, but it gets easier. And it's important. Most women will come back to me and say, "I had no idea what I was eating!"

alli

It's not that they were being dishonest with themselves, but they didn't think about that candy bar and the soda they had between lunch and dinner. Or the wine they had after work. Or that the portions they were served when they went out for dinner were huge. Or the late-night snack they had standing up in front of the fridge.

When you take the time to track it, you tend to start eating less.

[DR. GARY FOSTER]

food is family:
can't have one **without** the other

In my family we don't ask "How are you?" We ask "What should I bring?"
I know that they shouldn't have to go on a diet just because I do. When
the extended family gets together, it's impossible to eat right. There are
the big holidays. Don't even think about refusing seconds of my mom's
triple-baked cheese potatoes or pecan-molasses pie. The guilt she lays
on…it's easier to keep eating.

There are plenty of smaller occasions too. You can't attend summertime
barbeques at my brother's and then skip my sister-in-law's famous all-day
brunches. And don't forget manicotti at my mother-in-law's, with her
fist-sized homemade meatballs.

[you arrive with **one** dish, you leave with **six.**]

alli

Graduations, birthdays, whatever. The occasions may change, but the way we celebrate doesn't. We eat. And the celebration continues long after we've all gone home. At my family gatherings, you arrive with one dish, you leave with six, all brimming with leftovers.

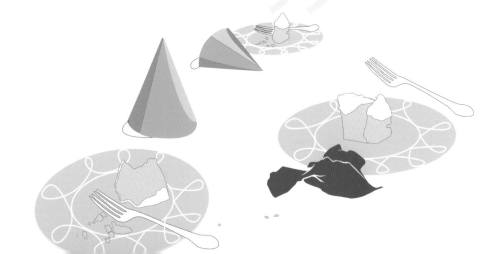

dr. foster weighs in:
be frank, speak firmly and bring a salad.

Family can be a huge issue. People tend to put caring for their family before caring for themselves. It's up to you to redirect your family's supportive instincts toward helping you achieve a healthy weight.

Let your family know you want to manage your weight. Have a serious, open conversation to solicit their support. Tell them that you aren't passing on seconds because you don't love them. You are doing it because you need to lose weight. Be honest and firm. Give them specific examples of how they can help: "Please eat the doughnuts in another room."

And when they honor your requests, be appreciative: "Thank you for picking up a salad instead of pizza."

Before you get together with the whole group, enlist the support of your spouse or partner. Ask them to back you up.

When everyone starts eating, try to revel in the conversation as much as the food. Suggest a walk after you eat. Bring a low-fat dish.

Don't tell yourself that it will be easier to like yourself when you lose weight. It will be easier to lose weight when you like yourself.

get out of your own way

7 things to get you started
here are my final thoughts.

"When people come to me, they talk about the pain of being overweight," says Dr. Foster. "They're embarrassed to participate in the mother-daughter softball tournament, or they can't walk up a flight of stairs anymore without getting breathless. They feel bad.

I tell them there is no quick fix, no magic pill. There never will be. Weight control is hard work, but it is doable. And self care is the key. It all comes back to that. You have to commit to taking the time for yourself."

alli

Where to begin? Dr. Foster offers simple ways to get started:

1 Keep a food diary. Know what you are eating.

2 Write down manageable goals. Instead of "I will lose three sizes by bathing suit season," try "I will eat a healthy, low-fat breakfast and lunch this week."

3 Begin an exercise program. Walk a block. Half a block if that's all you can tackle right now.

4 Reach out. You need the support of family and friends. Talk to them about what you are doing.

5 Go with a plan, not an empty promise. Don't vow, "I will eat less and be more active." Get specific. Say, "I will walk for 10 minutes today and eat fruit as my mid-afternoon snack."

6 Nobody's perfect. You will make mistakes. Don't ignore them, but don't beat yourself up over them. Forgive yourself, learn from what happened, and move on.

7 Focus on the process. This isn't a race. Don't approach it as a hard charge toward a finish line. This is a change in your lifestyle. Take it at a pace you can maintain and live with.

final tips

from gary foster, ph.d.

expect mistakes

prepare

rede

be

honest

don't be afraid

be prepared

One of the most successful strategies to losing weight is to plan and prepare meals and snacks ahead of time. Eating right takes more time than eating wrong. To do it right, you must take the time.

the way to weigh

Weigh yourself regularly, once a week, under the same conditions. Don't be afraid of the scale. And don't jump to conclusions if you weigh yourself five times a day. Keep track over weeks and months to understand the results.

learn from mistakes

You're only human. Expect mistakes. Don't focus on feelings of guilt or failure. What matters is what you do next. Ask yourself what happened. Be specific and honest. Then, rededicate yourself to staying on track.

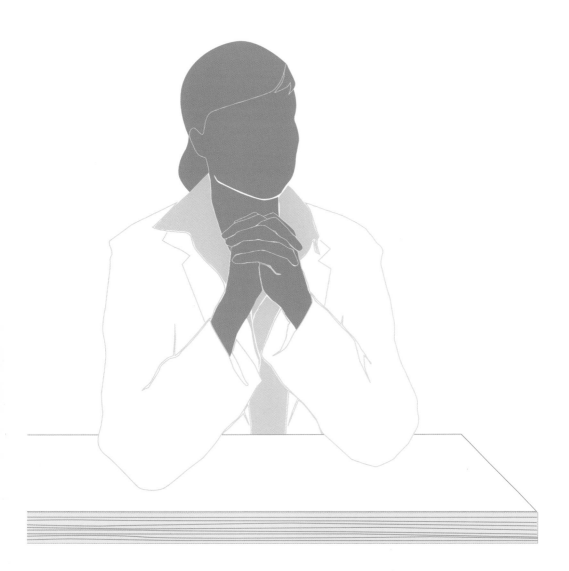

by **Caroline Apovian, M.D.,** director of the Center for Nutrition
and Weight Management at Boston Medical Center

fact or fiction?

Dr. Caroline Apovian answers 20 questions to separate fact from
fiction and help you recognize the reality of weight loss.

You know a lot about the outside of your body, but how much do
you know about how it works on the inside? How do cravings work?
What about low-carb and other fad diets? And what's the truth
about metabolism?

In this chapter, Dr. Caroline Apovian gives straight answers to 20 common
questions about weight loss. Read on as she cuts through the hype and
misinformation, offering facts about hormones, cravings, water and more.
Losing weight isn't as scary when you're armed with knowledge of how
your body works.

20 questions
with Dr. Apovian

1 **Why is it so hard for me to lose weight and other people can eat whatever they want and stay skinny?**

The short answer is: everybody and every body is different. Your genes, your environment, diet and physical activity are all related, so there is not just one equation for everyone. The truth is that although some people are genetically predisposed to be thin, there are very few people who can eat whatever they want without gaining weight.

2 **What about metabolism? Is there something I can take to increase mine?**

You can increase it, but not by taking anything. Your metabolism is correlated to the amount of muscle you have. The more muscle you have, the higher your metabolic rate. There are many ways to build muscle, even at home. Try lifting weights, using resistance bands or practicing yoga. But you have to do it regularly for maximum impact.

3 Do men burn calories faster than women? They seem to lose weight so much more quickly than women.

This relates to metabolism. Calories are units of energy used by the body. How many calories your body burns just to function is called your basal metabolic rate. Biologically, men tend to have more muscle than women. So yes, since men tend to have more muscle, and more muscle means a higher metabolism, men are predisposed to burn calories faster than women.

4 What about hormones? Do they play a role?

Yes, and again, it's related to metabolism. When you restrict calories and increase activity, hormones like leptin signal the body to reduce the metabolic rate and increase hunger signals. It's a survival reaction to protect fat stores. This is especially true for women, whose biological design requires more fat to protect the growth of a fetus. These hormones are also one reason people trying to lose weight have such a hard time—before your body adjusts to a lower caloric rate, it tries to get you to eat more.

fact or fiction?

5 But I've always heard that when you eat less, your stomach shrinks. Shouldn't that stop the hunger pangs?

Without gastric bypass surgery, your stomach won't ever actually get smaller. But after you maintain a lower weight for months, your body adjusts and the brain will receive a different pattern of signals. The result is that your body won't require as many calories to feel full. Your body will sense an environment where food is scarce and will adapt to this.

6 What can I do when I feel like I'm starving?

You should never feel like you're starving while you're trying to lose weight. If you're hungry in between meals, snack on vegetables and/or lean protein foods such as turkey slices. Protein is more filling than simple carbohydrates. Remember that you should eat until you're satisfied, never full. If you avoid stuffing yourself during meals, you'll likely avoid feelings of starvation later on.

alli

7 What about cravings? I yearn for the bad stuff—
candy, chips, fried anything. What can I do?

A craving is your body's way of asking for certain
nutrients. If your body needs salt, you might crave pickles.
An ice cream craving could be a request for calcium.
The key is to satisfy your cravings without over-indulging.
If you find that you're always craving chocolate, keep
low-calorie, low-fat chocolate treats on hand, or divide
your favorite chocolate treat into smaller portions and eat
only one portion per day. For example, you could make a
no sugar, low-fat hot chocolate for 50 calories.

8 Low-cal chocolate to stave off a craving for real
chocolate? I'm skeptical.

If you start eating healthier foods, after a while you will
begin to crave them. Incorporate healthier foods slowly
and with foods you already like (broccoli and cheese,
carrots and dip), and focus on finding healthy, low-fat,
low-calorie foods that you enjoy. Don't try to force yourself
to eat certain foods just because you think you should.

quick **tip**

**Manage your
cravings** before
they turn into
a night of
overeating.

45

fact or fiction?

[often people feel hungry and **eat...**

9   Is there anything I can do to prevent cravings?

Sure—try drinking water. Often people feel hungry and eat, when really, they are just thirsty. Drinking 8 glasses of water a day is not critical for weight loss, but it does play a big role in avoiding cravings. Water fills you up and doesn't have the calories found in soda and juice.

10   Some of my friends have lost weight on low-carb or no-carb diets. Is this the best way to lose weight?

Low-carb diets can produce significant weight loss in a short amount of time, because they maximize water loss in your body. The reduction in carbs produces less insulin, resulting in a loss of water and salt retention. Water loss equals weight loss. The problem is that it is very difficult to maintain low and no-carb diets over time. And once you introduce carbs back into your diet, the weight is likely to return.

alli

11 **Well, what about diets that require you to eat only one thing, like the Grapefruit Diet or Cabbage Soup Diet. Do they work?**

Like the low-carb regimes, these restrictive diets are designed to jumpstart weight loss by promoting water loss. And let's face it, who wants to eat only one type of food the rest of their life?

12 **But water weight is still weight. If I'm losing it, that's a good thing, right?**

Severely restricted diets could deprive the body of necessary nutrients. That's definitely not a good thing. Plus, extremely restrictive diets are unrealistic to maintain, even for a couple of weeks. Dieters usually end up gaining more weight than they originally lost. A balanced, reduced-calorie, low-fat diet is the healthiest approach to long-term weight loss.

when they are really just **thirsty.**]

quick **tip**

Make a chart to track your 8 glasses of water each day.

47

fact or fiction?

13 Wouldn't it be more effective if I just cut my calorie intake in half right from the start? That way, I'd lose real weight—not just water weight—fast.

No. Restricting calories too much, too fast, doesn't work. You not only deprive your body of important nutrients, but you set yourself up for a huge appetite and cravings that can lead to food binges.

14 Okay. What about my parents? If they were fat, am I destined to be fat as well?

While genetics play a big role, our environment and our habits also have a lot to do with our weight. If your parents were fat, can you be thin? Yes. Is it likely to be more difficult for you than your friend who has thin parents? Yes, but focus on what you can control. Come to terms with the fact that you may need to work harder and prepare for the challenge.

alli

15 Good fat, bad fat, trans fat, saturated and unsaturated fat— I'm confused. Wouldn't it be simpler if I just cut out all fat?

No. Cutting out all fat would extremely restrict food choices. Luckily, all fats are not created equal. Unsaturated fats (olive oil, canola oil, nuts, seeds and avocados) are "good" fats, but only in moderation. Stay away from saturated and trans fats (found in fatty meats and many processed foods) as much as you can. These fats raise cholesterol levels and increase your risk of heart disease. The alli program recommends limiting meals to 30% fat per meal, regardless of what kind of fat you're eating. That's an average of about 15 grams of fat per meal.

16 I've been yo-yo dieting since I can remember. Have I permanently slowed down my metabolism?

No. Gaining and losing weight in a "yo-yo" diet cycle doesn't slow your metabolism. That's a myth. Remember, metabolism is correlated to the amount of muscle you have. And increasing your physical activity rate will have a positive effect on your metabolism.

fact or fiction?

[if fad diets and miracle devices **worked…**

17 **What about age and shifting hormones? Doesn't that always mean "middle age spread"?**

No. "Middle age spread" doesn't have to be a fact written in stone. Age and shifting hormones don't slow your metabolism—losing muscle mass does. And there is a correlation between aging and losing muscle mass. If you find that as you age you are getting less physical activity, try to step it up a bit.

18 **So weight gain's not inevitable with aging?**

No, it's not. You have a choice. With a structured program of aerobic and strength training, people who are getting older can maximize their efforts to keep as much muscle mass as they can, and deter the middle age spread of fat.

alli

19 Are there any real, lasting benefits to weight loss other than the obvious—you look better?

Absolutely. By staying physically active and committing to a healthy diet, not only can you get a trimmed-down body, but you will make your heart healthier, have a lower risk of diabetes and improve your sexual functions.

20 Any final thoughts?

If fad diets and miracle devices worked, everyone would be thin and healthy. Weight gain isn't inevitable. Weight loss isn't easy, but the truth is that, at any point in your life, it's not too late to succeed.

everyone would be **thin** and **healthy.**]

final words
with Dr. Apovian

Dr. Apovian is right—weight loss isn't easy. You have to be committed to the hard work it takes to lose the weight, and the hard work it takes to keep it off. Knowing all of the science behind weight loss can help.

Every body is different, but everybody can do something to lose weight. Knowing that our metabolism is related to our amount of muscle mass is key to understanding the bigger role physical activity can play in weight loss. And it validates why we need to increase our amount of physical activity as we get older.

[at any point in your life...

alli

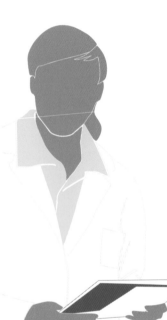

You know the cornerstone of a healthy weight loss program: principles of behavior change, eating reduced-calorie, low-fat meals, and understanding the human body. If you're ready to honestly commit to these principles, turn the page.

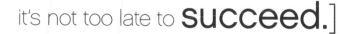

it's not too late to **succeed.**]

final tips

from caroline apovian, m.d.

stick to it
you decide
enviro
manage cra

think about what
commitment means

To prepare for weight loss success, you really need to think about what it will take and if it's something that you're willing to do. If you decide to do it right, make the decision permanently and stick to it.

satisfy cravings
without overeating

Cravings build up over time, leading to unhealthy binges. Manage your cravings with small servings to stay on track.

create a good environment

You may not be able to control your genes, but you can control your environment. Surround yourself with healthy food and don't put yourself in situations where you know you will overeat.

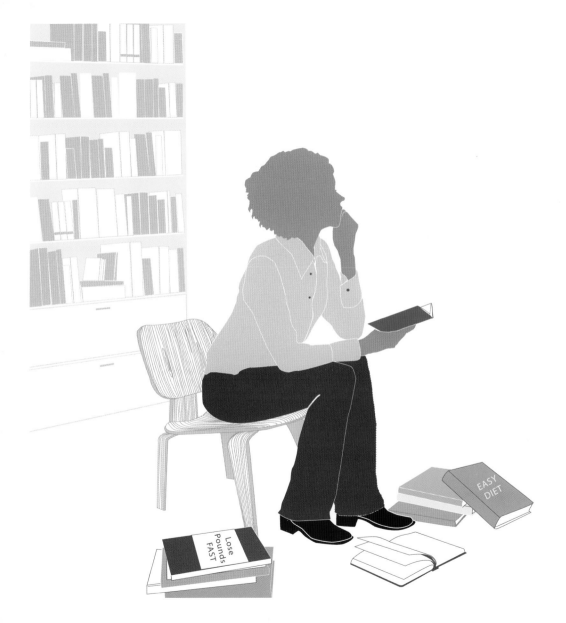

understanding alli

You're probably used to reading big, bold claims from other weight loss products that promise unbelievable results, so alli may come as a surprise to you. We're not going to tell you how easy it is to lose weight. Because it's not easy; it takes hard work and commitment.

But, if you follow the alli program and the advice in this book, you'll be well on your way to losing weight and losing it for good. We believe in what we've created with alli—that it can help you lose even more weight if you're willing to commit to eating reduced-calorie, low-fat meals.

[if you **aren't ready** to take responsibility...

alli is a 60 mg orlistat capsule. But what we've been researching and creating is more than just a pill. It's a complete program that will give you individually tailored support to increase your chances of succeeding. We're here to give you advice on changing behaviors, nutritional guidance, and the support to lose weight and live a healthier life. But only if you're ready.

Those who have been successful with orlistat, the active ingredient in alli, have been dedicated to changing their eating and activity habits. They know it's not a magic pill. They've experienced treatment effects and they know losing weight is hard work.

alli

alli is not for everyone, but alli is an option. The bottom line is this: if you aren't ready to make a commitment, we don't want you to buy it. If you are ready to take responsibility, alli can help you lose 50% more weight than dieting alone.

59

quick **tip**

Be honest with yourself. If you aren't ready to change how you eat, you aren't ready for alli.

we **don't want** you to buy alli.]

what is alli?

alli isn't just another product for you to buy. alli is a program: a pill with a plan. This program requires a commitment to living your life in a new way.

alli is the only FDA-approved, over-the-counter weight loss aid. The pill works by preventing your body from absorbing some of the fat you eat. The plan is individually tailored and works by providing you with education, tools, support, and incentives to help you succeed. That's big news.

alli

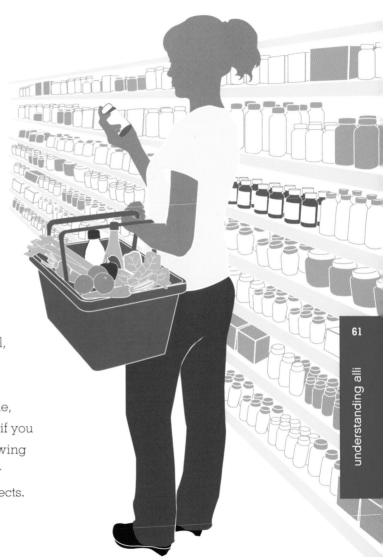

But alli isn't a miracle pill, and it won't guarantee overnight success. It can help you achieve sensible, gradual weight loss. But if you aren't committed to following the program, you'll likely experience treatment effects.

who is ready
for alli?

Are you ready for alli? Are you ready to change what you eat?
Are you ready to change your behavior?

alli is not for you if you're looking for a quick fix or if you only want
to lose weight to change things on the outside. It's also not for you if
you use food to cope with stress. You have to know that losing weight
is hard work, and it's going to take planning and dedication.

alli requires eating reduced-calorie, low-fat meals and physical activity,
and is for people who are committed to losing weight and doing it right
this time. You must be 18 or older, and overweight.

After you read more about alli, take the quiz on page 70 to test your alli IQ.

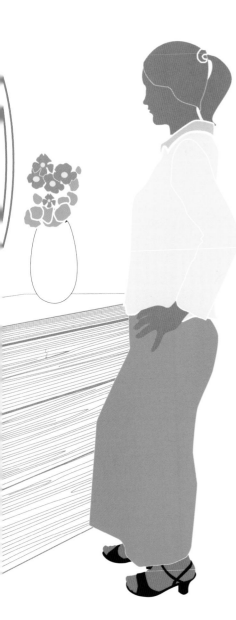

[alli is not a **quick fix.**]

Important:

Make sure you read and follow all of the
alli label directions, warnings, and all other
enclosed materials. As with every medication,
pay special attention to the warning and "do
not use" statements before you purchase and
use the alli weight loss aid.

how does
alli work?

You're probably curious about what alli does in your body and if it is safe. Here's how it works:

Part of the food you eat is fat. Naturally occurring enzymes in your intestines break down the fat from food, so your body can absorb it. The active ingredient in an alli capsule is a 60 mg dose of orlistat. Orlistat prevents the enzymes in your intestines from digesting about one-fourth of the fat you eat.

Undigested fat and calories cannot be absorbed and are eliminated from your body. Unlike some other weight loss products, alli only works in your digestive tract. It's not systemic and won't affect your brain or heart.

[results depend on a **reduced-calorie,**

allī

how much
can i lose?

If you are ready for the commitment, alli can help you lose 50% more weight than dieting alone. What does that mean in actual pounds? For every ten pounds you lose through a healthy lifestyle, alli will help you take off five more. Of course, results will vary from person to person, and will also depend on how closely you stick to a reduced-calorie, low-fat menu.

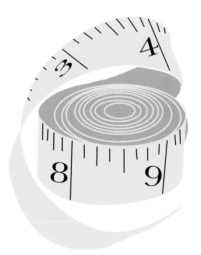

low-fat lifestyle.]

is alli
safe?

Yes, alli is safe. It is non-systemic and not absorbed into your bloodstream. alli only works in your digestive tract without affecting your brain or heart like some other weight loss products. This means no sleeplessness, jitters or increased heart rate. These findings are supported by extensive clinical testing. alli is the only over-the-counter weight loss aid approved by the FDA.

You must read and follow all label instructions before using alli. The information in the Drug Facts label will help ensure that the alli program is right for you, and that you get the maximum benefit from using alli capsules.

[alli will **not affect** your **heart rate.**]

alli

lose weight,
not nutrition

Taking a multivitamin every day is important for good nutrition when trying to lose weight.

It's especially important if you take alli, because alli reduces the absorption of some fat-soluble vitamins and beta-carotene. Take a multivitamin that has vitamins A, D, E, K and beta-carotene, once daily at bedtime, to ensure adequate vitamin absorption.

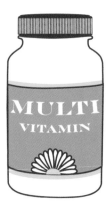

quick **tip**

Change your eating habits gradually so you can sustain them over the long term.

67

understanding alli

what about
side effects?

Unlike most weight loss products, alli has very few side effects because your body minimally absorbs the active ingredient. The main side effect occurs when you eat a meal with too much fat while taking alli. If so much fat is blocked that your stool can't absorb it, you might have side effects. We call them "treatment effects," and they can include loose or more frequent stools that may be hard to control, or gas with an oily discharge. The excess fat that passes out of your body isn't harmful, but you should be prepared for the possibility of it happening. In fact, you may recognize it as something that looks like the oil on top of a pizza. Treatment effects should be lessened if you stick to reduced-calorie, low-fat meals that average 15 grams of fat per meal.

alli   [treatment effects are **up to you.**]

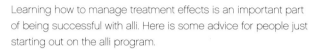

real tips for managing treatment effects

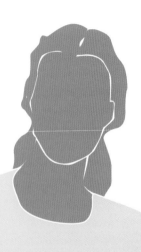

Learning how to manage treatment effects is an important part of being successful with alli. Here is some advice for people just starting out on the alli program.

- No one likes experiencing treatment effects, but they might keep you honest and avoid anything questionable for fat content. If you think of it like that, alli can act like a security guard for your late night cravings.

- Give yourself time to adjust. Starting the alli program when you have some time away from work will help you know what to expect.

- You can't "save fat grams" from lunch and "spend them" at dinner. Spread your daily fat gram allowance over the whole day.

- You may feel an urgent need to go to the bathroom. Until you have a sense of your treatment effects, it's probably a smart idea to wear dark pants, and bring a change of clothes with you to work.

- You may not usually get gassy, but it's a possibility when you take alli. The bathroom is really the only place to go when that happens.

- You can use a food journal to recognize what foods can lead to treatment effects. For example, writing it down may help you learn that marinara sauce is a better option than Alfredo sauce.

understanding alli

test
your alli
IQ

how much do you really know about fat?

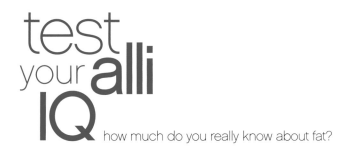

Part of being successful with the alli program is making smart food choices. Take the quiz to see how much you really know about weight loss and nutrition. Read all three choices and then circle the answer that best describes what you really think.

alli

1 How many Oreos® would you have to eat to gain a pound?
(There are 51 cookies in a package.)

    a. 33

    b. 66

    c. 99

2 A pound of fat is approximately the size of a _____.

    a. golf ball

    b. tennis ball

    c. softball

3 Which description contains the least fat?

    a. reduced fat

    b. low fat

    c. light

4 How many calories are in a pound of body fat?

    a. 1,500

    b. 2,500

    c. 3,500

5 What amount of peanut butter contains 16 grams of fat?

    a. 2 tablespoons

    b. 4 tablespoons

    c. ½ cup

....

6 Which fajita ingredient adds the most fat?

    a. 1 ounce of sour cream

    b. 1 ounce of cheddar cheese

    c. 1 chicken breast

....

7 Is eating six ounces of fresh tuna cooked with a tablespoon of olive oil a good choice with the alli program?

    a. yes, fish is healthy and you're avoiding butter

    b. no, this meal is too fatty for the alli program

    c. yes, olive oil contains the good kind of fat

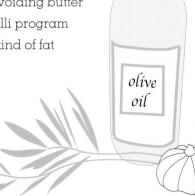

olive oil

8 A three-ounce serving of chicken is:

   a. a chicken breast and drumstick

   b. the size of a deck of playing cards

   c. the size of this book

....

9 One of the best predictors of successful weight loss is:

   a. keeping a food journal

   b. buying exercise equipment

   c. level of motivation

....

10 Adults are encouraged to take at least 10,000 steps a day to stay active. About how many miles is that?

   a. 1 mile

   b. 2.5 miles

   c. 4 miles

answers: 1) b 2) c 3) b 4) c 5) a 6) b 7) b 8) b 9) a 10) c

find out
your alli IQ

Check your answers and add how many questions you answered correctly. If your total was:

0-3 **You've taken the first steps to learning about choosing low-fat options.** You know the basics, but it might be helpful to pay more attention to food labels. For the alli program to help you succeed, you may need to change the way you think about eating and losing weight. Remember, if you cannot commit to the entire program, you'll experience treatment effects. We don't want you to buy alli until you're ready. For support—including help setting goals, healthier recipes to try, and more—visit my**alli**.com.

4-7 **You've done your homework when it comes to making smart choices.** Hopefully this quiz has opened your eyes and provided some helpful information. Being aware of serving sizes and fat content are essential to achieving success with the alli program. Remember, there is no halfway with alli. You have to be 100% committed. For additional insights and support to help you get ready, visit my**alli**.com.

8-10 **You understand a lot about low-fat eating.** That will help you make smart food choices, if you choose to follow the alli program. But there's more to it than just having the knowledge—you'll need to keep yourself on track. You can succeed if you commit to following the alli program, read all the materials in the alli starter kit, and visit my**alli**.com for regular support.

quick **tip**

It's easier to lose weight with the support of friends. Tell your friends to go to my**alli**.com and test their alli IQ.

support
keeps you going

Losing weight is easier with support. That's why the alli program includes an individually tailored online plan called my**alli**plan. my**alli**plan offers free support for up to 12 months, and was developed by nutritional and weight management experts who understand the struggle to lose weight.

After purchasing alli, you can access this innovative support program 24 hours a day at my**alli**.com.

when you register with my**alli**plan, you receive:

- A customized online action plan

- Personalized e-mails that deliver lessons about meal planning, managing hunger, dealing with setbacks, and making the food and lifestyle changes to help you succeed

- Menus and shopping lists

- A variety of online tools to record your food and lifestyle information

- Connection to a network of other alli users

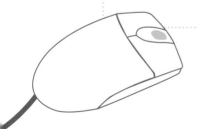

quick **tip**

You don't have to do this on your own. Use the tailored support from my**alli**plan to stay on track.

understanding alli

final **tips**

you are in charge
stay focused
positive infl

alli is only an option

You can lose weight following the advice in this book, without taking alli. If you decide to follow the alli program, you must make an extra commitment to avoid treatment effects.

support is not optional

Whether it's your friends, family, or just my**alli**.com, support is an essential part of losing weight. The more positive influences the better.

take responsibility

You are in charge of whether or not you will lose weight. Stay focused and understand that your efforts determine your results.

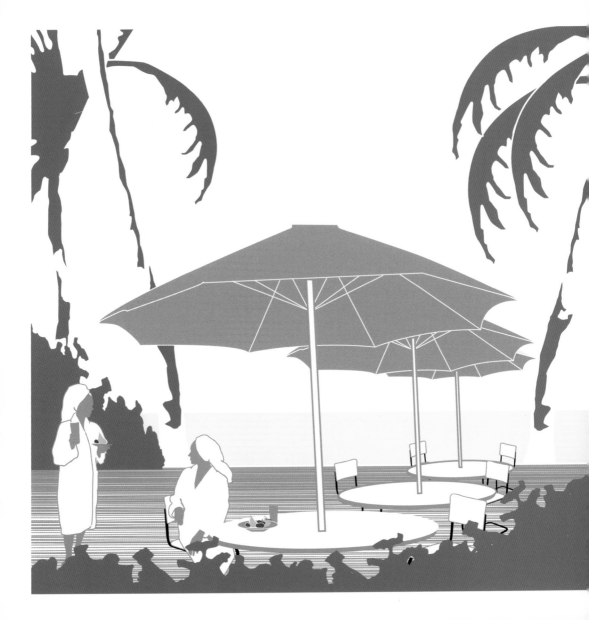

by Kathleen Daelemans
founder of Café Kula, author and television host

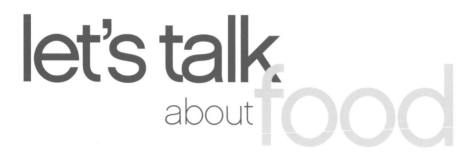

let's talk
about food

Chef Kathleen shares her stories, beliefs, and some of her amazing low-fat recipes.

Fourteen years ago, I was presented with an opportunity that changed my life. I was a chef working in San Francisco, and I lived for food. I ate like a size 22, and I was a size 22. I was in the kitchen all day, experimenting with new recipes—butter, cream cheese frosting, oils, more butter and choice cuts of meat. I made a mean hollandaise sauce, too.

There were times I thought about losing weight, but never did anything about it. I never had a reason to change. I worked hard. My work was food. Let's face it: my whole life was food. Heavy, rich and satisfying.

[i truly believe **food** is our **first line of**

After making a name for myself in the industry, another job offer came. The chance to launch a restaurant of my own. In Hawaii! At one of the world's most luxurious hotels. Whoa. Sounds great, right? What's the catch? I would be cooking for spa guests.

Spa cuisine? I wasn't exactly used to preparing or eating food that was spa-friendly. I decided to take a second look at food. I still wanted yummy and amazing, but I needed to find new methods and a new list of ingredients.

I started building a menu around the freshest fruits and vegetables and grilled or broiled lean cuts of meat. I became inspired. I changed the way I was preparing my own meals. With all of the big changes I was making, I committed to making the biggest one of all: losing weight for good.

and the best **medicine**

alli

defense...

I can't tell you that it was easy, but an amazing thing did happen. At first, pounds started dropping. Encouraged by that, I became more active. I felt great. Then, I started dropping dress sizes. That felt even better (and justified fun shopping sprees with my sister). But best of all, I really enjoyed the low-fat food I was preparing. On top of that: I felt fantastic and was full of energy.

I'm proud to say that through hard work and commitment, I lost 75 pounds, and I have kept it off for over 13 years. And you know what? My food is still extraordinary, delicious and satisfying.

we can prescribe for one another.]

quick **tip**

Eating low-fat doesn't mean eating low-flavor. Make the commitment to keeping your meals healthy and delicious.

let's talk about food

food for thought
what I learned to be true for me

I lived in denial, so I ate in denial. I thought nothing of having three bowls of sugary cereal with whole milk for breakfast. Ice cream as a mid-morning snack was perfectly reasonable. Vending machines and drive-thrus were frequent destinations.

I started taking weight off by changing my eating habits and focusing on portion size. It was then that I came up with my three culinary Ps to weight loss success: Portions, Preparation and Perseverance.

portions: It's easy to leave one bite behind, make a burger one ounce smaller and leave some of the milkshake in the glass. I was losing weight and gaining confidence. I made the decision to keep going.

So, I weaned myself down to normal portions. Size 10 portions. Not the teensy portions listed on some food labels, but what I consider to be normal and healthy for me and my body. I didn't do this overnight. I did it one food item at a time, one meal at a time, one day at a time.

preparation: Let's face it—you are in total control of what goes into your mouth and your grocery cart. Set yourself up to succeed by stocking your kitchen with foods you'd be proud to have broadcast on national television. If you'd be embarrassed by something, get rid of it.

Make sure that "whatever happens to be available" is good for your body. Because human nature dictates if something is there, we'll eat it.

perseverance: Coming from a world of indulgent, rich and fatty foods, did I have dark chocolate meltdowns along the way? You betcha! Do I still have binge-y moments? Yep. But I don't give myself permission to turn an oversized bowl of ice cream into a day of non-stop eating.

Take things one trip to the market at a time, one stint in front of the stove at a time, one meal at a time, one forkful at a time. Think about every bite you put into your mouth. Make it a good one. Watch what you eat and keep doing it. You can do this!

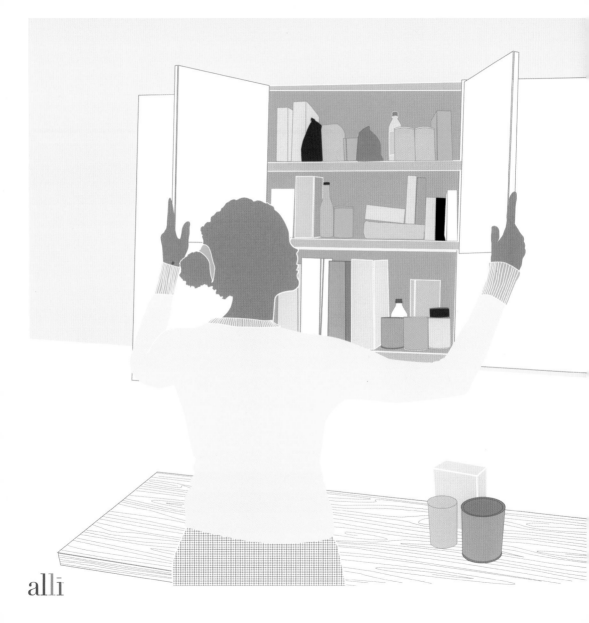

alli

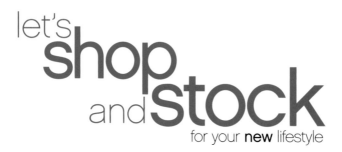

let's shop and stock
for your **new** lifestyle

I'm still tempted to eat the same high-calorie foods I love, but I don't stock them in the house anymore. If I have ice cream in the house, I will eat it. When it's gone, I can't blame it on the kids, the dog or my siblings. It's all me. Every single calorie and fat gram is mine to wear or work off.

Creating distance between the foods I cannot resist has helped me lose the weight and keep it off. For me, it's ice cream; yours might be chips, cookies, whatever. If it is bad for you, don't allow it around you.

let's be
honest

1 You don't need a nutritionist to walk into your house and point out the good, the bad and the evil. Just listen to your inner voice and use your common sense. Imagine a home economics teacher discussing the nutritional value of the item in question with a class of impressionable, young children. If you honestly believe Mrs. Healthy Heart would approve of the food you're debating, leave it on the shelf.

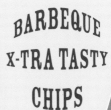

BARBEQUE
X-TRA TASTY
CHIPS

alli

2. **Discuss the plusses and minuses of each item. Think about how you might trade up.** If you're looking at a bag of wheat crackers that have sugar and hydrogenated oils, consider the portion listed on the label and the amount you usually consume in a single sitting. Multiply the number of servings in the box by the number of calories per serving. Are they the right choice for you or your family? Are those calories really worth keeping in your life? And on your hips?

3. **Donate the unwanted items that are unopened to your local food pantry or shelter.** Also, please give yourself permission to throw the rest away. A little waste now makes for a lot less waist later on.

let's talk about food

[CHEF KATHLEEN DAELEMANS]

let's go
shopping

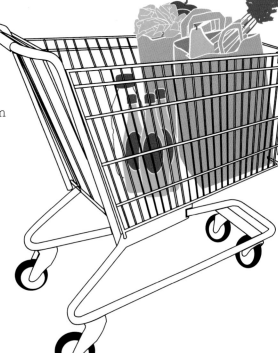

1 If you don't see it, you won't buy it.
Don't cruise the cereal, candy, soda or cookie aisles. Avoid stores with end aisle displays stacked top to bottom with the newest junk food.

2 I do all my shopping at a normal supermarket.
You might enjoy checking out a specialty health or international grocery store.

alli

3 Carry a permanent list of staples—it will save you time—and make it in order of the store's layout. Pick five easy dinner recipes, check their ingredients against your inventory, and go from there.

4 You are shopping for a week. Just looking at your cart will tell how committed you are. You should have seven days worth of vegetables, fruits, lean protein and whole grains.

quick **tip**

Try to get in and out of the grocery store in about **30 minutes.**

let's talk about food

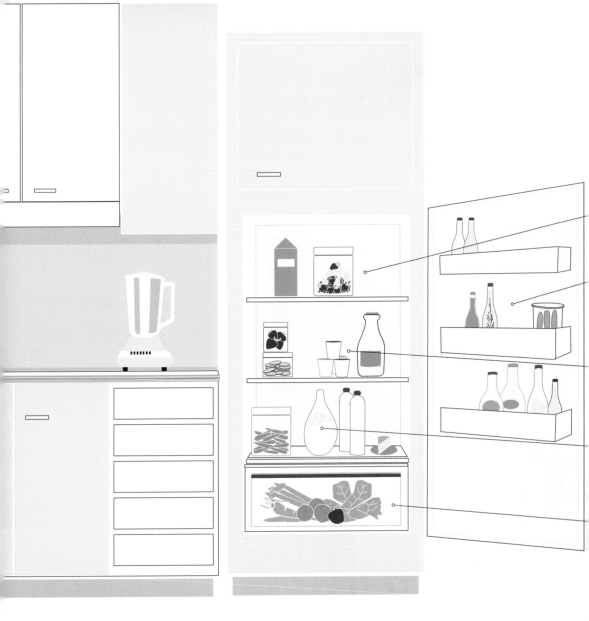

let's redo your
fridge

snacks : **eye candy:** Always have fresh fruit on hand for a snack—oranges, apples, cherries, berries and chunks of melon. Fresh fruit is affordable and delicious.

on the side : **condiments:** Hot sauce, low-sodium soy sauce and mustards.

make it pickled: Dills, kosher spears, and any pickled vegetable you like.

pepper it up: Cuisines from Mexican to Italian to Indian use peppers. Try poblanos, serranos and jalapeños to heat things up.

dairy : **low-fat dairy:** Skim milk, eggs and fat-free yogurt.

hold the cheese, please: Dry aged cheeses, like Parmesan, are satisfying—and go a long way. Avoid soft cheeses.

drinks : **water:** Adding lime or lemon adds more taste. Avoid juices high in sugar.

soda: If you have to have a soda, make it diet.

protein : **meat/fish:** Stock your fridge and freezer with pre-portioned servings of pork, beef, skinless chicken breasts, and fish. One serving size shouldn't be bigger than the size of a deck of cards.

let's talk about food

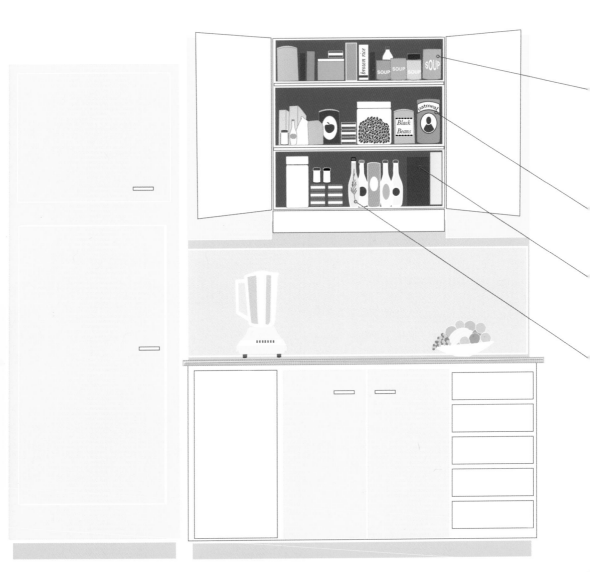

let's prime your
pantry

canned goods : canned soups: They're convenient. Just make sure they're low-sodium. Many are often two servings.

canned beans: Low-sodium chickpeas, black beans, white beans and non-fat, spicy refried beans.

canned tuna and chicken: Packed in water.

canned tomatoes: Low-sodium crushed, whole peeled plum, tomato paste and ground peeled.

good grains : grains: Brown rice, wild rice, flax meal, wheat germ and barley oats. Breads, pastas and tortillas should be whole grain.

cereal: Oatmeal. It's good for you without the sugar.

baking : basics: Whole wheat flour, all-purpose flour, baking soda and powder, kosher and iodized salt. Add some flavor—vanilla, almond, orange and lemon extracts.

seasoning : vinegars: Red, white, rice and balsamic.

oils: Dark sesame and extra virgin olive oil. But use sparingly; a tablespoon of oil usually contains 14 grams of fat.

spices and dried herbs: Fat-free and zero-prep flavor boosters.

quick **tip**

While following the alli program, you need to be **extremely careful with oils** to reduce the possibility of treatment effects.

let's talk about food

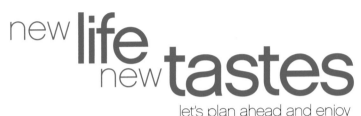

new life
new tastes

let's plan ahead and enjoy

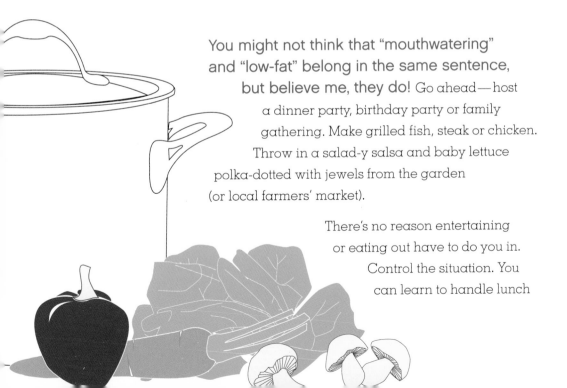

You might not think that "mouthwatering" and "low-fat" belong in the same sentence, but believe me, they do! Go ahead—host a dinner party, birthday party or family gathering. Make grilled fish, steak or chicken. Throw in a salad-y salsa and baby lettuce polka-dotted with jewels from the garden (or local farmers' market).

There's no reason entertaining or eating out have to do you in. Control the situation. You can learn to handle lunch

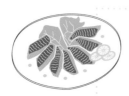

perfect dinner parties

- ☐ show-stopping ahi tuna with spicy napa cabbage salad
- ☐ chicken with quick citrus pan gravy
- ☐ baked pears with red currant jam

on the run, a quick meal after work, or impressing your friends—and still lose weight the healthy way.

hearty, healthy soups

- ☐ mushroom barley soup
- ☐ sausage, chickpea and sweet potato stew
- ☐ asian chicken noodle soup

On the following pages you'll find my favorite low-fat recipes for any occasion: entertaining, midweek meals, lunches and even five-minute meals for when you're in a hurry— or just plain tired from a long day.

5-minute meals

- ☐ mix and match to create quick, yummy meals

easy, everyday lunches

- ☐ 10 lunches to look forward to

- show-stopping ahi tuna with spicy napa cabbage salad
- chicken with quick citrus pan gravy
- baked pears with red currant jam

enjoy good food with good friends
perfect dinner parties

If you're having guests, turn to summery cookbooks for Thai, Japanese, Indian, Chinese, Mexican, California and Pacific Rim inspired recipes. A lot of the food served in hot climates is naturally healthy and low in fat. Choose recipes with short ingredient lists and items where the work is already done for you, like pre-grated vegetables.

There's a lot of flavor to be found in cilantro, lime, mint, hot sauces, soy sauce, etc.

alli

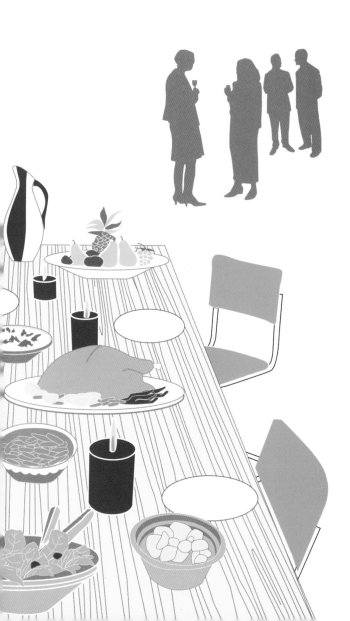

quick **tip**

When your guests compliment the meal as they leave, **surprise them with the news it was low-fat.**

let's talk about food

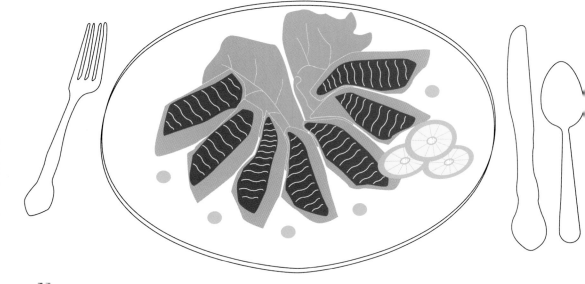

[CHEF KATHLEEN DAELEMANS]

[spend **more time** with your friends...

alli

show-stopping ahi tuna
with spicy napa cabbage salad

PREP TIME: 30 MIN I **COOK TIME:** 4 MIN I **SERVES** 4

- 2 tablespoons lime juice
- 1 ½ tablespoons fish sauce
- 1 teaspoon sugar
- 1 teaspoon sesame oil
- 1 medium napa cabbage
- 1 bag shredded carrots
- ½ cup basil leaves, torn into quarters
- ½ cup mint leaves, torn
- ½ cup cilantro leaves, roughly chopped
- 1 pound ahi tuna in one piece (ask for sashimi grade)
- coarse-grained salt and cracked black pepper
- 2 teaspoons sesame oil

1 In a large salad bowl, whisk together lime juice, fish sauce, sugar and sesame oil. Taste and adjust seasonings. Cut cabbage in half, lengthwise. Place cabbage, carrots, basil, mint and cilantro into the bowl with dressing. Toss to combine. Place a generous amount of salad on each of the four serving dishes.

2 Season fish with salt and pepper on both sides. Heat oil in a 12-inch, non-stick pan over medium-high heat. Add fish to pan and cook until rare, about 2 minutes per side. Alternatively, cook until done to your liking. Using a sharp carving knife, slice thin. Place equal amounts on each of the four salads. Garnish with sprigs of fresh cilantro and lime wedges.

and **less time** in your kitchen.]

quick **tip**

This dish is great with grilled or broiled shrimp, lightly pounded boneless, skinless chicken breast, or thinly sliced seared or grilled steak. **Think four ounces of protein per guest.**

101

let's talk about food

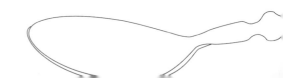

chicken with quick citrus pan gravy

PREP TIME: 10 MIN **I COOK TIME:** 10 MIN **I SERVES** 4-6

- 1 pound boneless, skinless chicken breast, lightly pounded
- coarse-grained salt and cracked black pepper
- 2 teaspoons olive oil
- 4 garlic cloves thinly sliced
- ½ cup orange juice
- 1 teaspoon fresh thyme leaves

1 Season chicken on both sides with salt and pepper. Cook chicken with olive oil and garlic over medium-high heat for 3-4 minutes per side until golden and tender.

2 Remove chicken and add orange juice to the garlic in the pan. Bring to a boil, add thyme. Reduce to a simmer until thick. Pour sauce over chicken and serve.

alli

baked pears with red currant jam

PREP TIME: 10 MIN **I COOK TIME:** 30 MIN **I SERVES** 4

I'd never eat or order baked pears anywhere, ever, because I always felt they were a cliché "diet" dessert. I couldn't imagine they'd taste good, let alone turn out to be sublime and a dish I loved so much I wanted to learn how to make it. They're really, really wonderful when you're in the mood for something warm and cozy, and they couldn't be easier to prepare.

- 3 tablespoons brown sugar
- ½ cup water
- 4 ripe pears, peeled, cut in half and cored
- 8 teaspoons red currant jam

1 Preheat oven to 425°. Whisk ½ cup warm water and brown sugar together in a 9 x 13 inch oven-proof baking dish. Stir sugar to dissolve. Place pears in a single layer in pan bottom and turn to coat with liquid.

2 Place in oven and cook, turning once at the halfway point, until pears are cooked through and soft, about 30 minutes.

3 Remove from oven, place a teaspoon of jam into the core of each pear and serve immediately.

forget your can opener
hearty, healthy soups

I rarely get through a 12-hour workday and think,
"Yippee, I get to go home and cook!" In a perfect world,
I'd open the front door and a butler would take my briefcase and coat,
hand me a glass of champagne, usher me to the dinner table, pull out
my chair, lift the sterling silver dome off my fine china, and recite the
ingredients and derivation of the meal in front of me. But let's face it: at
the end of the day what happens is, I walk in the door from work, throw
my stuff on the floor, grab a fork and stand in front of the refrigerator,
grazing from shelf to shelf until I'm full and satisfied. I've made peace
with this character flaw by stocking my freezer with reheat-and-eat
soups. On the weekends, when I have the time, I like to make a double
batch of a hearty soup, stew or chili.

alli

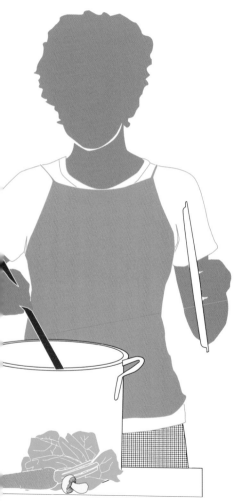

Then I divide leftovers into individual or family size servings and store them in the freezer for nights I'm too tired to cook. By planning ahead, you can have a dinner that's faster than fast food and a whole lot healthier and tastier, too.

quick **tip**

Kids love noodle soups. Try adding fun pasta shapes to make recipes even more family friendly.

let's talk about food

mushroom barley soup

PREP TIME: 20 MIN I **COOK TIME:** 90 MIN I **SERVES** 4-6

This calls for dried porcini mushrooms. If you don't have any, pick some up the next time you're out. They add a deep layer of rich flavor and of course, they're virtually calorie free. I wouldn't call for them in a recipe if the result wasn't worth it.

- 1 cup dried porcini mushrooms
- 2 slices thick-cut bacon, cut crosswise into thin strips, about ⅛ pound
- 1 small onion, finely chopped
- 1 small carrot, finely chopped
- 1 rib celery, finely chopped

- 1 cup pearl barley
- 8 cups water
- juice of one lemon
- ¼ cup loosely packed, grated parmesan cheese

1 Pour 2 cups warm water over mushrooms and let stand until softened, about 20 minutes. Heat a large soup pot over medium heat until hot, add bacon and cook until golden and starting to crisp, about 4 minutes. Add onions and a splash of water and cover. Reduce heat to medium and cook until onions have completely softened, about 10 minutes. Add carrots and celery and cook 5 minutes more or until just starting to turn tender.

2 Strain mushrooms, reserve one cup of their liquid. Dice mushrooms very fine and add to soup pot with their liquid. Add the water and bring to a boil. Add the barley, reduce to a simmer and cook, partially covered, stirring occasionally, until barley is tender, about one hour. Add lemon juice, taste and adjust seasonings with salt and pepper. Ladle into soup bowls and top each portion with a little bit of grated cheese.

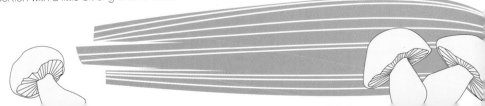

alli

sausage, chickpea and sweet potato stew

PREP TIME: 30 MIN **I COOK TIME:** 30 MIN **I SERVES** 6-8

This super-nutritious stew is out-of-this-world great. My dad, who is not a fan of anything healthy, would eat steak and potato gratin seven nights a week if he could get away with it. Every time I make this for him, miraculously, he asks for seconds.

- 2 teaspoons oil
- 1 small onion diced (can use frozen diced onions)
- 2 cloves minced garlic
- ½ pound low-fat Italian chicken sausage, casings removed
- 1 28-oz. can crushed tomatoes
- 3 cups low-sodium chicken broth
- 1 sweet potato, about 1 pound, peeled and diced into ½ inch chunks
- 1 teaspoon ground cumin

- 1 teaspoon fennel seeds crushed with the bottom of a heavy skillet
- 1 small squash such as buttercup, about 1 ½ pounds, peeled, seeded and diced (can use frozen diced squash or low-sodium squash soup, but fresh squash is the best!)
- 1 15-oz. can chickpeas, drained and rinsed
- coarse salt and cracked black pepper to taste

1 Heat oil in a large soup pot over medium-high heat. When hot but not smoking, add onion and garlic. Cook, uncovered, stirring every now and then, until onion has completely softened, one to two minutes. Add sausage and cook, breaking it apart with a spatula or spoon, until cooked through, two to three minutes.

2 Add tomatoes, broth, sweet potatoes, cumin, and fennel seeds. Bring to a boil, reduce to a simmer, and cook until sweet potato is almost done, about 10 minutes. Add squash and chickpeas and cook, uncovered, for 15 to 25 minutes more, until squash is fork-tender. Taste, adjust seasonings with salt and pepper, and serve.

let's talk about food

asian chicken noodle soup

PREP TIME: 20 MIN **| COOK TIME:** 20 MIN **| SERVES** 4

This is the first thing I make when I feel a cold coming on. The ginger and warm nutritious broth combined with the chili's heat seems to chase away my aches and fever and clears my sinuses. I truly believe food is our first line of defense and the best "medicine" we can prescribe for one another.

- 4 tablespoons low-sodium soy sauce
- 2 tablespoons mirin (rice wine)
- 2 teaspoons sesame oil (dark)
- 1 clove garlic, minced
- 2 tablespoons fresh ginger, minced
- 1 tablespoon sugar
- 4 tablespoons rice vinegar
- ½ teaspoon Vietnamese chili paste
- 8 cups chicken broth

- 12 ounces boneless, skinless chicken breast, cut crosswise into thin strips
- 4 cups Chinese vegetables or napa cabbage, chopped
- 1 5-oz. package of rice noodles, prepared according to packing directions
- ½ cup loosely packed, roughly chopped cilantro
- 6 scallions, thinly sliced on the bias, white and some green

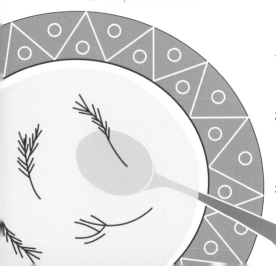

1 In a small, non-reactive bowl, whisk together soy sauce, mirin, 1 teaspoon sesame oil, garlic, ginger, sugar, vinegar and chili paste.

2 In a 3 quart soup pot, heat the broth, add soy sauce mixture, the chicken and the vegetables. Bring to a boil. Add remaining sesame oil. Taste and adjust seasonings.

3 Pour over prepared Chinese noodles. Garnish with cilantro and scallions.

ways to make these soups your own

Just because a recipe has a list of ingredients, doesn't mean they are set in stone. Get in the kitchen and experiment to see what combinations of ingredients give your soup that extra oomph. Feel free to mix and match and come up with your signature recipe.

soups	add flavor	add texture	add spice
mushroom barley soup	minced garlic	cubed, cooked potatoes	crushed red pepper flakes
asian chicken noodle soup	stir-fry sauce	steamed rice	garlic szechwan sauce
sausage, chickpea and sweet potato stew	parmesan cheese	chopped fresh spinach	louisiana-style hot sauce

let's talk about food

microwaves aren't just for making popcorn
5-minute meals

Make your microwave live up to its potential. Your microwave is not the best cooking tool you have in your kitchen. But when you're short on time, it gets the job done for steaming veggies or reheating already cooked meats. We're talking speedy and savory.

5-Minute Formula: A broiled, grilled or pan seared serving of lean protein, one or two microwave steamed veggies and a tossed salad. Are the meals five-star gourmet unique? Not so much. But with a little advanced planning, you can get dinner on the table in five minutes.

alli

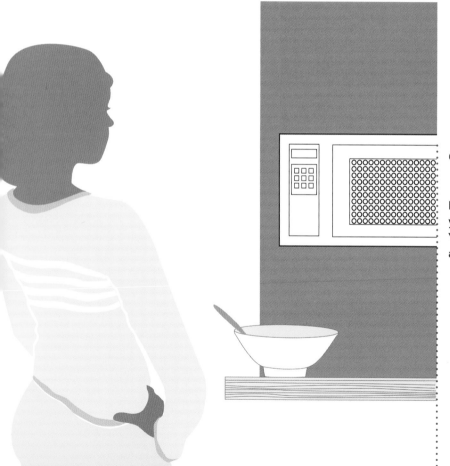

quick **tip**

Don't overcook your vegetables. **You'll lose flavor and texture.**

let's talk about food

mix and match to create quick, yummy meals

Pick one food from each category to follow the 5-minute formula:
protein + veggie + salad = a quick, delicious and healthy meal.

protein	veggies	salad
chicken	asparagus	arugula with lemon
white fish	peas	spicy carrot slaw
pork chops	green beans	iceberg with vinaigrette
flank steak	carrots	spinach with oranges
turkey breast	corn	mixed greens

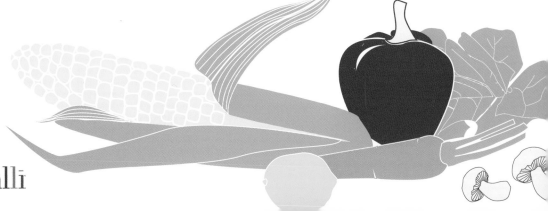

alli

example: chicken with asparagus and arugula

Here's a quick combination of protein, veggies and salad with delicious results:

1 Chicken: To prepare, lightly pound ¾ of a pound of boneless, skinless chicken breast (one piece). Season with salt and pepper. Heat 1 teaspoon oil in large nonstick pan; when hot but not smoking, add chicken and cook turning once until golden, about 3 minutes per side. Let stand 2 minutes. With a sharp knife, slice thinly and divide among four serving plates.

2 Asparagus: Place in baking dish with 2 tablespoons water. Cover loosely with plastic wrap. Cook on high or vegetable setting until done, about 2 to 3 minutes for one bunch. Toss with balsamic vinegar, salt and pepper. Divide among four plates.

3 Arugula with lemon: Arugula (about 4 cups to serve four) tossed with the juice of a lemon, a drizzle of olive oil (about 1 teaspoon) and a sprinkling of Parmesan cheese, about 2 tablespoons for four people.

it's quick food, not fast food

easy, everyday lunches

If you have to "make" lunch, chances are you won't. If all
you have to do is pack a lunch, chances are you will. Studies show
that we consume more calories when we eat out, between 100 and 1,000
more per meal!

Effortless Prep. Outrageous Meals. When you're planning menus for the
week, keep lunches in mind. Create lunch fixings by preparing extra. Grill
an extra chicken breast or an extra few ounces of lean steak or pork.

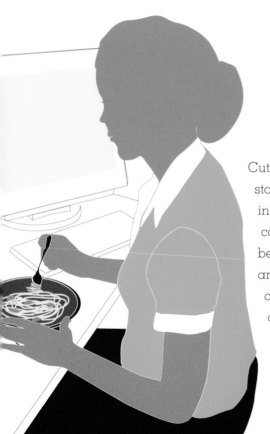

Cut the meat into strips, store in snack size bags in the freezer. Cabbage, carrot, fennel and beet slaws keep well and can turn a boring chicken wrap into a deeply satisfying lunch.

quick **tip**

Leftover cooked veggies can turn into a soup or chopped salad meal quicker than you can say **please pass the peppermill.**

let's talk about food

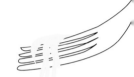

10 lunches
you will look forward to

1 leftover steamed veggies tossed with a can of tuna and low-fat salad dressing make an interesting salad to take to work.

2 leftover grilled chicken tossed with low-sodium, canned black beans, defrosted frozen mango chunks or unsweetened pineapple chunks and low-fat sesame dressing.

3 canned, low-sodium lentil soup with a generous dollop of zero fat Greek style yogurt, a squeeze of lime and a tablespoon of chopped cilantro.

4 leftover soba noodles with mandarin orange sections, baby spinach, chopped chicken and low-fat sesame honey dressing (2 teaspoons low-sodium soy sauce, 1 teaspoon rice vinegar, 1 teaspoon honey, 1 tablespoon fresh orange juice, ½ teaspoon sesame oil whisked together).

5 low-fat refried beans spread on a whole wheat tortilla with leftover brown rice and low-calorie tomato salsa.

alli

6 low-sodium butternut squash soup with canned chickpeas, a squeeze of fresh lemon juice and a tablespoon of chopped parsley.

7 hummus wrap ¼ cup prepared hummus (chickpea dip), 2 tablespoons prepared baba ganoush (eggplant dip), 2 ounces very thinly sliced leftover chicken or steak, wrapped in a whole wheat tortilla.

8 chopped vegetable salad roughly chopped leftover steamed vegetable medley (think frozen veggies steamed in the microwave) tossed with honey mustard dressing.

9 microwave or baked whole sweet potato (re-heated at work) topped with zero fat Greek style yogurt, a squeeze of fresh lime juice and a tablespoon of chopped cilantro.

10 reheat and eat leftover beef and veggie stir-fry Cook 4 ounces of thinly sliced chicken or steak with a teaspoon of peanut or sesame oil. Bring ¼ cup low-calorie bottled szechwan stir fry sauce and ¼ cup water to a boil. Add one bag frozen asian vegetable medley. Cook, stirring often until veggies are cooked through and well coated with sauce, about 5 minutes. Serve. Pack leftovers to go in microwave-safe containers, reheat and eat at lunchtime.

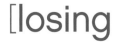

my final food for thought
10 things to always remember

I'm living proof that modest lifestyle changes can result in weight loss, a greater fitness level, and a lot of confidence.
In my wildest dreams, I never imagined I'd become a spa cuisine chef, let alone a weight loss success story, 75 pounds and counting. It took a lot of hard work and commitment, but I've never felt better.

The key is to realize this is your new life—your new low-fat lifestyle. Food is important. You should always enjoy what you're eating. Otherwise, it won't last. If you're ready, I know you can do this, too.

[losing

alli

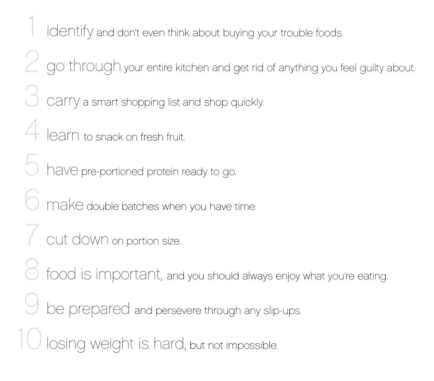

1 identify and don't even think about buying your trouble foods.

2 go through your entire kitchen and get rid of anything you feel guilty about.

3 carry a smart shopping list and shop quickly.

4 learn to snack on fresh fruit.

5 have pre-portioned protein ready to go.

6 make double batches when you have time.

7 cut down on portion size.

8 food is important, and you should always enjoy what you're eating.

9 be prepared and persevere through any slip-ups.

10 losing weight is hard, but not impossible.

weight is hard, but **not impossible.**]

final tips

from chef kathleen daelemans

plan a menu
stay engaged
accou
avoid empty

stay engaged

Keep living healthy in your thoughts every day. On days that you're not being physically active, you can plan a menu. You create accountability by keeping weight loss in your internal dialogue.

eat breakfast

Starting the day hungry sets you up to overeat later in the day. Studies show that people who eat breakfast are less likely to be obese. A healthy breakfast will stick with you.

eat well-balanced snacks

Make snacks that have both carbs and protein. Avoid empty calories. Choose foods that will fill you up and taste great.

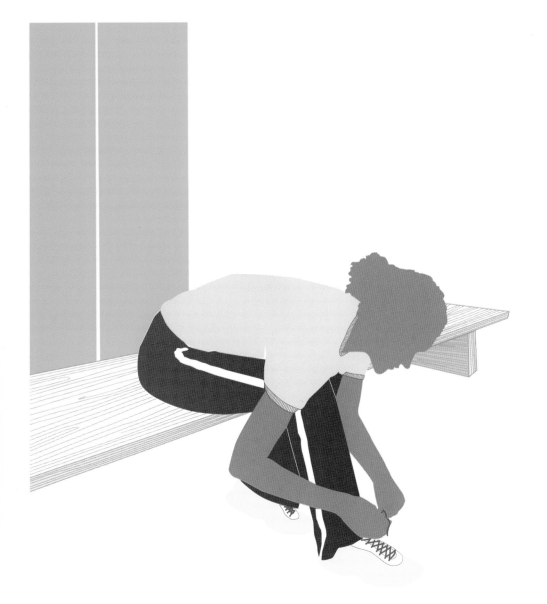

by Madelyn Fernstrom, Ph.D.
founder and director of the Weight Management
Center at the University of Pittsburgh Medical Center

let's get moving

Dr. Madelyn Fernstrom shares fun ways to add physical activity to your everyday life.

Now that you understand how important it is to eat reduced-calorie, low-fat meals, you can think about other ways to help you increase your weight loss. The alli program is certainly one of them. And when you add physical activity to the mix, you can lose even more.

You might be surprised how easy it is to add more activity to your day, and how easy it is to make being active fun—for you *and* your entire family. Here, Dr. Madelyn Fernstrom offers tips on how to incorporate activity into your life and burn extra calories doing the things you already do. She also offers ideas on how to make staying active a part of your life without sacrificing time with family and friends.

123

let's get moving

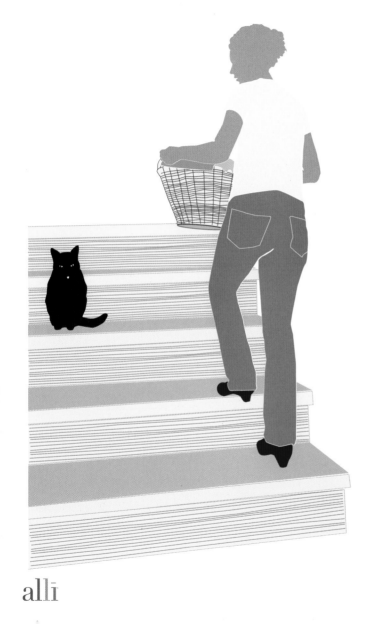
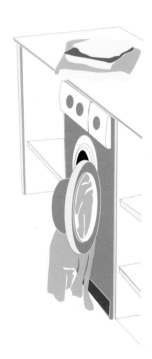

alli

burn
calories
without
exercising

Joining a gym or running for miles is great exercise. But it isn't the only way to get moving and burn some calories. Check out these tips for fun ways to stay active.

Sit down. Yes, sit. Turn on the TV if you want to. Just make sure you're sitting on an exercise ball (there are large ones, and smaller disc exercise balls that can fit on an office chair). The ball will make you sit up straight, and help strengthen your core muscles (including abdominal and back muscles). Remember, greater muscle mass means you burn calories more efficiently, and the increased muscle tone gives you a leaner look.

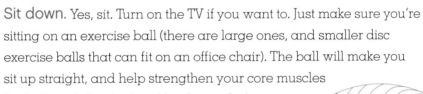

Stand up. If you're not using an exercise ball, stay on your feet. Even standing burns more calories than just sitting down. Try conducting a meeting or having conversations while standing. You might find that you're even more efficient on your feet.

Make a phone call. Gone are the days of being tethered to the phone with a twisted cord. Phones are mobile, so you can be, too. Whether you're at home or at the office, start walking around while you talk. Five 5-minute calls (or one long heart-to-heart talk) burn about 100 calories.

Deliver a message. Instead of sending e-mails or telephoning a co-worker down the hall or a neighbor across the street, deliver the message in person. You'll save time in the long run by getting an immediate answer. Acting as your own personal message service for 10 minutes a day burns about 50 extra calories a day, which can add up to 5 fewer pounds over a year.

Be (selectively) inefficient. Sure, we pride ourselves on being multitasking superheroes. But sometimes, it pays to be a little inefficient. Make extra trips up and down the stairs at home instead of trying to bring everything up at once. A load of laundry, the kids' toys, and an old coffee mug can each be brought up separately, turning 10 used calories into 30.

alli

6 Activity you can count on. Don't worry about finding time to get moving—make time by setting an alarm on your cell phone or watch. Set an alarm to go off three times a day and walk around for 10 minutes. No snoozing on this alarm. You'll get a half hour of walking each day without needing a huge block of time.

quick **tip**

It's easy to stay on the couch, but your body and mind always feel better after burning some calories.

129

let's get moving

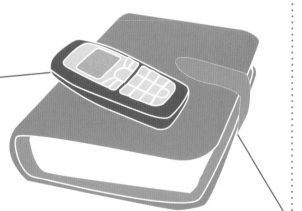

7 **Move to the beat.** You don't have to leave your house to stay active. Flip on the radio or some music videos and turn your living room into your own private dance floor. Dancing is a fun, easy way to burn calories. Plus, it's a natural stress-reliever.

8 **Take flights.** Stair climbing is one of the easiest calorie burners around. Ten minutes of stair climbing (about 10 flights) use up as many calories as a walk twice that long on a flat surface. Just beginning? Alternate the stairs and the elevator—get off one or two floors before your destination. And always walk up the escalator. (No free rides!)

9 Walk 'n' shop. When you get to the mall, take a lap around the perimeter before you start shopping. Every time you make a purchase, take another lap. You can count your steps by wearing a pedometer—every 2,500 steps is about a mile.

10 Add pounds you can remove at the end of the day. Put a few books in a small backpack and build up your strength while burning calories. Lugging around extra weight, even for an hour or two, also builds muscle. Use a small backpack to distribute weight evenly. If you're fatigued within several minutes, switch them to a stroller. Likewise, don't load up too much too fast in the backpack.

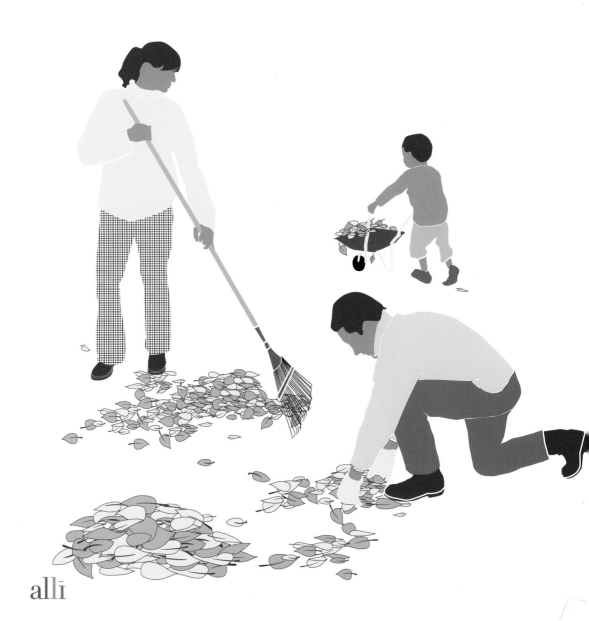
alli

connecting
with **friends**
and **family**

It's easy to think of being active as a lonesome pursuit. But a workout doesn't have to be at the expense of family time or a social life. Here are ways you can get fit while connecting with friends, family and co-workers.

1 Catch up with loved ones. Few of us have time to sit down together for a family dinner every night of the week. When the crunch is on, try a 10- to 20-minute walk with your family instead. These mini-hikes can be a great way to catch up on the daily family events. The destination doesn't matter; it's the together time that counts. As for dinner, make sandwiches or other portable foods ahead of time that everyone can grab after the walk.

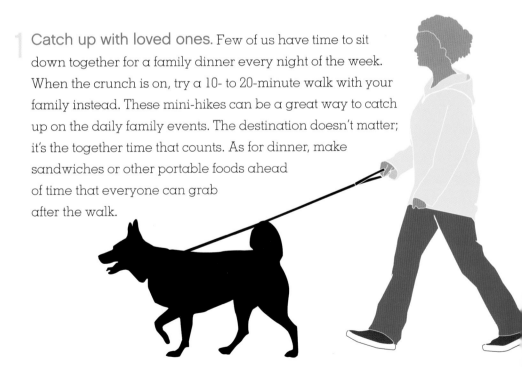

alli

2 **Jump for it.** You won't have to tell your family how many calories they will burn to get them to have fun on a trampoline. It's a stress-relieving way to stay active and enjoy some time outside. Or there are smaller, more affordable trampolines with handlebars designed to keep one person active and off the ground. These are easy on the joints and fun to do while watching TV or spending time with your family.

3 **Walk the dog.** Many of us delegate this task to children, spouses, or professional dog walkers. Do it yourself, once a day. Your dog will fall in love with you all over again. Better yet, bring the entire family along and take turns choosing the route.

4 **Get growing.** Gardening, whether it's a big yard or a few pots, is a great way to be active. Choose a friend who likes to garden, then spend time weeding and pruning throughout the season, and enjoy the beauty of a wonderful garden. For extra benefits, use a watering can instead of a garden hose: this burns calories from lifting weight and increased walking.

5 **Get framed.** Instead of dinner and a movie, why not bowl a few frames after you eat? Or choose bowling over a movie on a rainy day. It's a great stress-reliever, good physical activity, and a lot of fun. Many people start as occasional bowlers for family activity, and then find a friend for regular league participation.

6 Be a sport. Use half-time at your children's sports games to walk and chat with some of the other parents. It's just as easy as standing still and talking, but it gets you on your feet and might even help you meet more people.

7 Go play. Turn off the TV, shut down the computer, grab the kids and head for the playground. While it's fun to be an observer, try to minimize the bench-sitting. Push someone on a swing, or even swing yourself. Climb on the monkey bars, revisit the seesaw and check out the slide. And don't feel silly! Your children will be delighted, and you'll get your blood pumping.

Physical activity can help reduce lots of negative things, **from risk of heart disease to stress.**

let's get moving

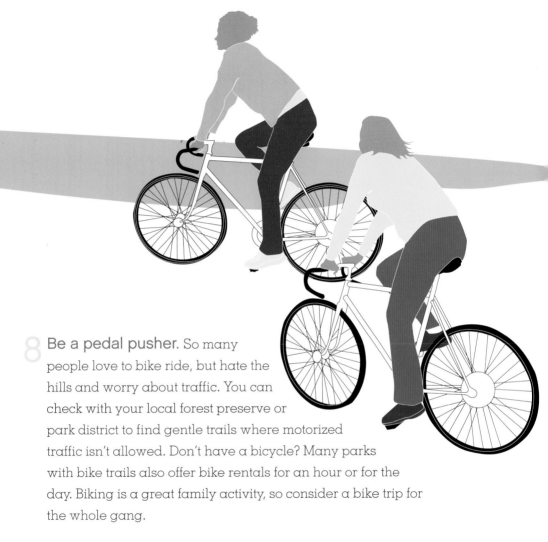

8 **Be a pedal pusher.** So many people love to bike ride, but hate the hills and worry about traffic. You can check with your local forest preserve or park district to find gentle trails where motorized traffic isn't allowed. Don't have a bicycle? Many parks with bike trails also offer bike rentals for an hour or for the day. Biking is a great family activity, so consider a bike trip for the whole gang.

alli

9 **Wash the car.** Choose a sunny day, grab some sponges and the hose, and head for the driveway. Whether you work alone or enlist a family member to help, you'll get a workout vacuuming the interior and scrubbing the exterior. Use plenty of good old-fashioned elbow grease and you'll get a workout and make your car sparkle. Bonus: you can use the money you would have spent at the carwash to splurge on a personal indulgence—a new lipstick, a juicy bestseller or a pedicure.

Get moving and **your body will continue to burn calories** hours later.

let's get moving

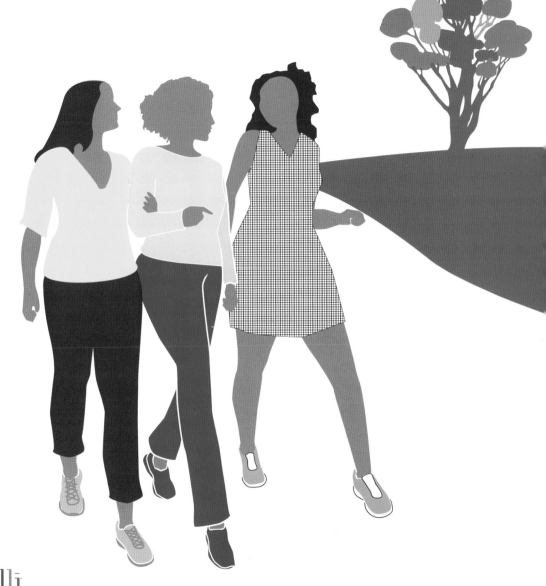

alli

dr. madelyn fernstrom's closing thought
keep moving every day

Eventually, as your new lifestyle takes root and your energy level increases, you'll be able to ramp up your activity even more. The key at the beginning is to make small changes that fit easily into your life. You don't want to become overwhelmed. You also don't want to burn yourself out or wake up aching. Remember: every journey starts with a single step. Keep taking them. Be consistent and you will succeed.

final tips

from madelyn fernstrom, ph.d.

keep it up

stay active

food

count your

wear a pedometer

Counting your steps is a fun way to make sure you stay active. Get at least 10,000 steps a day and you're on your way.

if you bite, write

Keeping a food journal is extremely helpful for many reasons. It keeps you thinking about what you eat, helps you to avoid silly calories, and gives you records to study to interpret your weight loss results.

making moving fun

If you don't enjoy something, you can't keep it up forever. Find ways to stay active every day doing things you like.

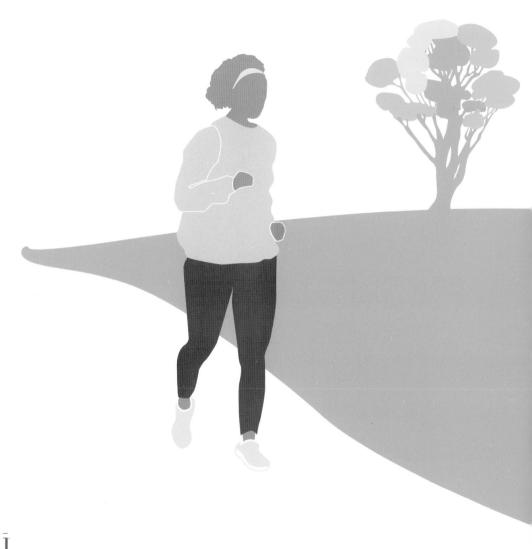

allī

Now you know that your success isn't up to alli, it's up to you. The program works best when you put in the hard work. If you can make the commitment to the program, it can help you meet your goal to lose weight and keep it off.

Start by making a commitment to yourself and getting your kitchen ready with the foods that will help you succeed. Make sure you're giving yourself time to prepare these foods and time to eat them. Also, be sure to find time to relax and time to be physically active. Not only will physical activity help reduce stress that can lead to cravings, it will also help you lose more weight and gain more muscle—which you now know helps you burn even more fat.

You're going to want to keep this book handy and read it over again when you have questions, or perhaps when you want to try one of Chef Kathleen's delicious low-fat recipes. You might want to share this book with a friend who may or may not be ready for alli. You can also go online to my**alli**.com and start reading all of the great support information.

You know that alli is not a magic pill. And you know that you need to follow the rules of the program to avoid treatment effects. We hope you realize that you're worth it and that you can do this for you.

You can count on alli to give you support and connect you with others who have committed to alli. If you're ready, the support

[the first step is often the

alli

begins as soon as you purchase the alli starter pack. It includes all the tools and information you'll need to be successful with the alli program.

Share your story and your success with others at my**alli**.com, where you can get encouragement and advice as well. It's an exciting journey, and we're with you every step of the way. The first step is often the hardest to make, but often the most rewarding.

If you're not ready yet, we'll be here for you when you are.

But if you *are* ready, it's time to buy the alli starter pack. It's time to stop losing your mind trying and start losing weight successfully.

hardest to make.]

contributors

dr. gary foster

Gary Foster, Ph.D., is the director for the Center for Obesity Research and Education and a professor at the Temple University School of Medicine. He has a doctorate in psychology from Temple and has authored or co-authored more than 100 articles and two books on the treatment and causes of obesity. As a clinician, he has worked with thousands of people over the years, helping them to lead healthier lives.

dr. caroline apovian

Caroline Apovian, M.D., is the director of the Center for Nutrition and Weight Management at Boston Medical Center, a nutritional consultant for NASA, and a professor at the Boston University School of Medicine. Dr. Apovian devotes her clinical time to seeing patients who want to lose weight, anywhere from 10 to 200 pounds and more. She has treated thousands of patients over her career as a physician nutrition specialist. She also spends part of her time conducting clinical research on fat cells and new ways to help people lose weight.

kathleen daelemans

Kathleen Daelemans is a professional chef who focuses on healthy eating. While opening a new restaurant in Hawaii, she dropped 75 pounds and went from a size 22 to a size 8. Daelemans has a best selling cookbook and has hosted a cooking show, demonstrating that healthy eating does not have to be time consuming, unsavory or difficult. When it comes to healthy cooking and eating, Daelemans is "her own best advertisement."

dr. madelyn fernstrom

Madelyn Fernstrom, Ph.D., is the founder and the director of the Weight Management Center at the University of Pittsburgh Medical Center. She has a doctorate from the Massachusetts Institute of Technology where she studied biochemistry, metabolism and neuropharmacology. She has treated thousands of patients struggling with weight issues, basing her work on the conviction that obesity is a chronic disease that can be managed.

The contents and advice contained within this book are based on the contributors' understanding of current science and their own expertise. They have been compensated for their time, but the opinions and advice shared are theirs alone.

Are you ready to commit?

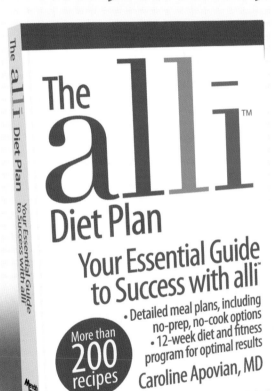

An important tool for anyone interested in losing weight with alli™.

- More than 200 delicious recipes

- Meal plans including no-cook, no-prep options

- Detailed section on eating out

- Low-intensity, fat-burning and toning fitness program to maximize results

- Long-term guide to maintaining your weight loss and tips on how to stay on track

The information and guidance provided in this publication are not intended to be a substitute
for medical advice. The reader should first consult with his/her healthcare practitioner before
commencing a new exercise regimen or if he/she has any medical concerns regarding his/her
diet, weight or general health. As with all medications, **alli** weight loss aid should not be taken
without first reading the entire product label and then only when following the directions for use.
The contents of this book are neither a substitute for nor an addition to the **alli** label directions.
The author and publisher expressly disclaim responsibility for any adverse effects arising
directly or indirectly from information contained in this book.

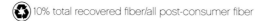 10% total recovered fiber/all post-consumer fiber

alli, my**alli**.com, my**alli**plan, alli Shuttle, and various design elements are trademarks of GlaxoSmithKline.
Copyright © GlaxoSmithKline Healthcare 2007

For information about permission to reproduce selections from this book, write to Permissions,
GlaxoSmithKline, 1000 GSK Drive, Moon Township, PA 15108

Library of Congress Cataloguing-in-Publication Data is available.
ISBN-10: 0-9779604-2-0
ISBN-13: 978-0-9779604-2-2
Printed in the United States of America

losing weight

isn't easy

nothing worth it ever is